HOW TO GO PALEO

For Natural and Healthy Weight Loss

by Kitty Browne

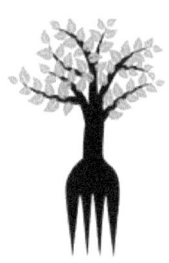

Kitty Browne Multimedia
Denver, CO

www.KittyBrowne.com

Table of Contents

Millions of Years in the Making

Henry St. John, the philosopher whose work inspired not only Voltaire but also the movement towards democracy in the United States, once told us that "history is philosophy teaching by example and also by warning."

Now, he probably wasn't thinking about diet plans when he made that great statement, but the sentiment is so universal that it's worked its way into nutritionist's hearts regardless.

Here's why: imagine, if you will, a cavewoman. We'll call her Reeja. Now, Reeja's job in life (apart from reproduction) was pretty simple; she was a gatherer. On any given day, Reeja would sally forth into the world. She would scrabble about in the dirt, trying to find the camas roots and sort them out from, say, the similar-in-all-but-one-respect "death camas" roots. She knew which berries to harvest, which tree's fruit was safe.

Now, she'd never think about grass seed. Grasses provided no nutritional value, and their seeds were hard and tough; not good to eat. Reeja was highly skilled at knowing which plants were edible. She hadn't yet figured out that if you took that grass seed and bashed it between two rocks, you would get a powder that, when mixed with water and heated up over fire, turned into delicious bread. No, Reeja was concerned with plants that were *edible,* not plants that could be *made edible* with processing.

Wild potatoes, onions, fruits, vegetables; these were Reeja's go-to. On top of that, she'd be picking up grubs, snails, bugs, as small protein sources. If she were really, fabulously lucky, one of the men in the village would have killed some larger animal: rabbit, squirrel, or (fingers crossed) deer, elk, boar, or bison.

Again, if Reeja was lucky, her group of cavepeople would have discovered/stolen fire. With that fire, she could heat up whatever she had that was big enough to jam onto a stick and hold over the fire. If she was really, really creative she would heat up a flat rock in the fire, and then use that to heat some of the other things she had gathered.

This was the maximum extent to which Reeja would go to convert the hunted and gathered food into the eaten food. She was simply not technologically advanced enough to do anything else with it.

I'm going to take a moment here to note that anthropologists are still bickering over gender roles and social structure. This isn't that book; I know that I'm using commonly-held gender stereotypes here, but please, bear with me. The point here is this: Reeja's efforts were combined with similar efforts of cavepeople everywhere, and were the only thing to feed and sustain our ancestors.

Imagine, for a moment, Reeja's reaction if she could simply walk into a modern grocery store. The volume and variety of fruits and vegetables that can be found in just one aisle of the grocery store would take her weeks or even months to gather, and even then she wouldn't be able to keep it all from going bad. She'd at least know what to do with them, though: eat them.

The meat aisle would be strange, but not entirely unfamiliar. The idea that you can just go somewhere and get meat without having to run it down and often risk your own health or safety would be completely foreign. Buying just enough meat to use before it went rancid would be something of a new concept, and the refrigeration units we have would confuse and terrify poor Reeja, but she'd be able to look at the meat and know what to do with it. Eat it. Maybe heat it up first, but eat it.

Now let's think about the *rest* of the store. We've got two sections in which Reeja is, at least, solidly grounded. Everywhere else is powders, oils, sauces, baked goods, and non-water beverages with strange colors and even stranger textures. The sheer level of *processing* that has gone into these items would, to Reeja, place them into the category of not-food.

For tens of thousands years, Reeja and her companions determined the diet of proto-humanity. Evolution being what it is, and medicine being what it *wasn't,* those people whose bodies had adapted to deal with the menu placed before them by Reeja lived. Those people who couldn't thrive when presented with Reeja's menu were culled from the herd. The invisible, Darwinian hand selected the fittest and bred them into…us.

Our bodies were forged not by companies like Nabisco and Western Family, but by gatherers like Reeja. Agriculture has only been around for ten, maybe fifteen thousand years. When compared to the development of our digestive and metabolic systems, this is but the blink of an eye. The modern grocery store, with its preserved, packaged food and oils, has been around for an even shorter period, perhaps a hundred years at best.

It should not, then, come as a surprise that science has told us that Reeja's diet may actually be healthier for us than the diet of excess and luxury our modern convenience has provided us with. That confused, terrified reaction Reeja had when looking at our modern store? *Your body has the same reaction.*

Enter the Paleo Diet, a diet reaching back to humanity's roots in small, hunter-gather societies, before the rise of agriculture and domesticated animals and livestock. It's based around the principles that simple, natural food like what our ancestors ate is still the best food to nourish our bodies to this day.

Now, just because you eat naturally, doesn't mean that you have to eat "rabbit food" all of the time. While our ancestors in the Paleolithic era did eat a lot of root vegetables, berries and leafy greens, foods that occur naturally also include game animals, fish, eggs, mushrooms, and honey, just to name a few.

It's not very likely that many people in the present day have the time or resources to spend their whole day hunting and gathering like back then, but we don't have to. Remember, there were entire sections of the grocery store where Reeja would have been confused by the refrigeration units, but perfectly at home with the food contained therein.

Reeja also didn't have a lot of tools at her disposal. She might have a spear or a harpoon, but other more sophisticated hunting weapons such as a bow and arrow hadn't been invented yet. And because the Paleolithic era is before the agricultural revolution, she doesn't have cereal crops, such as wheat, oats, or corn available either. Cows weren't domesticated until about 11,000 years ago, so Bessie the milk cow was still several thousand years away.

This means the Paleo diet focuses on eating fresh, locally available, organic fruits, vegetables, nuts, meats and fish, and avoiding refined or processed foods, such as flour, sugar, salt, cheese, and most oils. Basically, if you could feasibly find a food while on a camping trip, it's perfectly fine to eat on this diet. But if it requires complex aging, curing, refining, or domesticating animals to eat, that food wouldn't be included in the foods our bodies actually evolved to digest.

The Paleo Diet is based off of knowledge that even though Reeja lived many, many centuries ago, the genetic structure that makes up both her and people today really hasn't changed. Because Reeja and her family could only eat what was available in the wild, humans are genetically more equipped to eat those types of naturally found in a hunting-gathering situation. Foods which can contribute to digestive problems such as lactose-intolerance, Celiac Disease, and Type II Diabetes are all foods which Reeja didn't feed her family.

From what archaeologists and other scientists have been able to find out about Reeja and her contemporaries, she fed her family a diet rich in protein and fiber, but low in carbohydrates. The exact percentage of protein in Reeja's menu is still a matter for debate among dieticians, but everyone agrees that Reeja's diet was much lower in salts, sugars and other carbohydrates than the everyday modern diet.

In this book, we're going to explore the methods and benefits of bringing your diet back into this most ancient form of eating. We'll take a look at how you, in your everyday life, can eat just like Reeja did, and we'll take a look at why it may very well be the healthiest option available.

How Does 'Going Paleo' Work?

Ok, so we've covered an interesting hypothetical about the Paleo diet, but it's time to dive into hard science. What is it about Reeja's way of eating that leads to weight loss and overall improvement in health? Is this another fad diet, or is this really a lifestyle that will change your body in a positive way?

Evolution

The recent new advances in DNA research in the last few years have led to some startling discoveries– not the least of which is how little our DNA has changed from that of Reeja and our Paleolithic ancestors. Analysis of the DNA in Paleolithic bones have shown that at least physiologically, the changes in the basic building blocks of humanity really have been negligible in the intervening years.

When you really think about it though, that's not that shocking. It's only been a few thousand years, or around 333 generations, since the agricultural revolution changed the way humans had been surviving and eating for millions of years.

The industrial revolution occurred even more recently, and hasn't made any significant dent on our DNA at all. Our DNA is still identical to our relations that lived before our modern proliferation of cities and mass-produced food.

Pre-Industrial people's DNA, Reeja's DNA and our DNA is all basically interchangeable.

Once we understand that, the other science behind the Paleo diet begins to fall into place. When researchers looked an indigenous people in Africa or the Aleutians who still live a hunting and gathering lifestyle, the rate of the digestive diseases that plague Western Civilization is remarkably low. These populations have a very low incidence of high blood pressure, heart disease, diabetes, or obesity. (Eaton, 119-123) This can't just be explained away by saying they're eating less than their western contemporaries. In most cases this isn't true. What is different is the types of foods they are eating. They are consuming the same foods that our bodies have evolved over millions of years to be able to digest and they are meeting more of the accepted vitamin and nutrient standards set by researchers and dieticians! (Kligler, 139-140)

Carbohydrate Consumption

"Low-carb" has been a catchphrase amongst dieters for at least a solid decade now. That's because our bodies get carbohydrates in (even ones that aren't sugar to begin with), and convert them into sugars. This cycle is one of the biggest contributing factors to being unable to lose weight or gaining weight while on a low calorie but high carbohydrate diet. Reeja's diet didn't use these complex carbohydrates, so her body wasn't constantly on this high to low blood sugar cycle.

Of course, sugars are good, fast energy for the body. We're hard-wired to *like* sugar, because sugar gives us energy.

In Reeja's day, calories were a *good* thing, but Reeja couldn't process grains into flour. Over the years, humanity has added more and more carbohydrates to our diet because that's what we are inclined to eat. Bread, pasta, rice, cakes, oatmeal; all of these are high-carbohydrate substances that we *love* to eat.

Reeja would have loved them too, if she'd known how to make them.

Reeja didn't have many sources of pure sugar available in her environment, either. Most of the sugars she ate would have been simple fructose present in fruits or vegetables, which are much easier for our bodies to process. If she was really lucky she might come across a beehive and get a small amount of honey. The gallon jars of honey that we get from modern apiaries would cause her jaw to hit the ground.

In most loaves of bread there are multiple things the human body was not evolved to use- grain, milk, butter, refined sugars, and vegetable oils. With all the ingredients that are more difficult for the body to digest, it's not surprising that most people have trouble losing weight on high carbohydrate, low protein diets.

Furthermore, the high carbohydrate diet is actually more likely to lead to other health problems due its tendency to cause the person to have a high glycemic index for a prolonged period of time. A high glycemic has been linked to an increased risk heart problems and the loss of artery elasticity.

We've condensed carbs into smaller and smaller packages, allowing us to eat more and more of them. This, of course, means we've enabled ourselves in consuming more and more calories.

The Paleo diet avoids the spikes in blood sugar and insulin production inherent in eating bread products. Grains, even the supposed "healthier" whole grains, cause a cycle that pushes blood sugars high and then allows them to crash a few hours later.

This sugar crash results in the feeling hunger, fatigue, and eating more, even if your caloric needs have already been met. To get through the sugar crash, the most common reaction is grab another grain-based food, which is what caused the sugar crash in the first place, causing the cycle to repeat.

By switching to a diet high in protein, natural fruits and vegetables and nuts, it simultaneously cuts out a lot of the empty fat calories that most Western societies eat in bread products without even really thinking about it.

Returning to Reeja's diet means stepping away from that high-and-crash cycle that carbohydrate consumption gives us. The desire for carbs built into our bodies was put there before we could obtain carbs in such abundance; it's now pumping carbs into us at a rate our bodies simply cannot handle. The result of going back to Reeja's way of eating is, therefore, to limit that abundance. By doing that, we've naturally dropped the bottom out from our calorie consumption. Weight loss, health, and resistance to type II diabetes follows from that.

Fat Consumption

We *love* caloric foods, and little makes food taste better than fat. That makes sense; fat is a storage container for energy; it's there to pack as many calories into as little space as possible. Remember, Reeja *wanted* calories; as a result, we're programmed to think of fat as just wonderful.

Everything I said about carbohydrates can just as easily be applied to fats, but exponentially more so. We've got lards, vegetable oils, and butter aplenty in our diet. The entire dairy section of the grocery store, a place entirely foreign to Reeja (with the exception of the occasional lucky egg), is a vessel for fats.

Almost every meal we make begins by putting oil in something. "Grease and flour a 9" x 13" baking pan" is one of the most common instructions on the back of baking boxes these days.

Now, Reeja's diet was not without fat. If she could get her hands on some meat or some fish, she was going to eat it. But it was without *refined* fat. That is to say, Reeja never went out of her way to distill fat away from its original value.

No cooking oil, shortening, or butter could be found in her cave; if she was eating fat, she was getting a high dose of protein along with it. Current science shows that protein actually helps the body to feel full and also cues the body's metabolism to produce more energy. At the same time, this type of diet ups the "good fats" being consumed from fish such as Omega 3 and monounsaturated fats from nuts or avocados.

As a result, the types of fat you're consuming on the Paleo diet are far healthier.

The amount of fat you're consuming is far less, because you're avoiding all of the *refined* fats. Less and healthier fat means less calories and a better cardiovascular system.

As a result, the Paleo diet comes out far ahead for fat consumption than just about any diet out there.

But I thought milk does a body good?

"Drink your milk."

This is a command that has become a mantra in the mouths of mothers worldwide. Before we can even speak to question it, we are told that milk is a good, healthy substance for us. It's a part of our daily culture.

Don't get me wrong here. Milk *is* a pretty amazing substance.

Think of its original, natural purpose; it's there to provide everything a growing calf needs to get bigger and begin functioning on its own. It's calcium, vitamins and calories in the form of a blend of acid and fat. An infant animal can absorb vast amounts of nutrition from this substance, and for good reason; it's not getting nutrition anywhere else.

But here the story takes a bit of a turn.

Adults simply don't need that many saturated fat calories, and we certainly don't need it in beverage form. We don't need the lactic acid; we're producing enough of that as it is on our own. Milk's a substance designed to make a small animal a lot bigger.

When adults consume it...well, it tends to make us a lot bigger.

The fact of the matter is, Reeja and all her kin never thought to milk a cow, but they still managed to survive. The human body isn't built to process milk as an adult, and it's in almost everything.

Here's the thing: calcium can only be absorbed into the body when it's in the body in a soluble form. The consumption of dairy actually nets an acidic balance in the body that leads to more calcium being lost than absorbed, even though cheeses and yogurts often have a high level of calcium in their original form.

Fruits and vegetables have a more alkaline base, and so are more likely to net a less acidic, more balanced solution in the body which leads to more calcium being absorbed than is lost. This actually, for an adult, makes fruits and vegetables a more viable source of calcium than the dairy.

Vegetables such as spinach are actually a much more effective source of calcium than dairy. A lot of the calcium in milk actually passes through the human body. Calcium needs other vitamins present in order to be absorbed, and is actually present in milk in lower quantities than spinach, kale, collard greens, or almonds.

So don't worry about the lack of milk. Your body was built to run without it; it will do just fine avoiding dairy.

Vitamins and other health benefits

Reeja's body took what it could from the food it was presented with, and generated the rest on its own. Those kind of Reeja's that couldn't survive that way didn't last long enough to become our ancestors.

It should come as little shock, then, that the focus on eating natural foods means that the Paleo diet contains more naturally occurring antioxidant and anti-inflammatory vitamins and minerals than the standard Western diet, helping to protect heart and immune health. All the B vitamins, Vitamin A, and a whole host of other positive factors come into play when we're talking about the paleo diet.

The fruits and vegetables in the Paleo diet will also get you more vitamins than a standard diet

The only vitamin that the traditional Paleo diet may not provide enough of is Vitamin D.

When exposed to the sun the cholesterol in people's skin turns to vitamin D, so this wouldn't have been a problem for Reeja and her contemporaries, but if you have a job that keeps you indoors, you may want to take a vitamin D supplement. Western diets usually get their vitamin D from fortified dairy products. This usually only supplies about 60% of the recommended level of vitamin D, but it is more than the Paleo diet by itself provides from food alone.

Our body is designed to benefit from the foods found in our natural environment, because that is how humanity survived for millions of years. Our DNA is not designed to work with highly refined foods such as sugar, grains, dairy, and complex fats and oils.

Studies have shown that low calorie, high protein, low carbohydrate diets are better for losing weight and keeping it off than low calorie low protein, high carbohydrate diets. (Journal of Nutrition and Environmental Medicine, 149-60)

Getting Started with the Paleo Diet

The Paleo diet is actually really simple to follow in your day-to-day life. If it's not something you could imagine Reeja finding on one of her foraging or hunting trips, it is not Paleo. To translate into more modern terms, if it's not something you could find out on a camping trip in the wild, and catch or pick up to eat with minimal processing, then it's probably not included.

That goes double for things you would never find in the wild, such as refined oils, sugars and grain products. For example, you would never find rolled oats in a form that could easily be eaten in the wild, so they aren't included in the Paleo Pantry.

The rule of thumb is this: think of Reeja going down the grocery aisle and picking foods that would be considered "edible" to her. Certain areas of the store, she'd figure out easily. Other items she simply would not recognize as food. If she would have problems figuring out that the item is food, chances are the digestive system you inherited from her is going to have the same problems.

One caveat on that, is that you still want to pick vegetables that are non-starchy, since those convert into sugars in the body and have reduced dietary fiber. (Joulwan)

The major foods included in the Paleo diet are:

- Lean meats and game animals

- Eggs

- Fish

- Mushrooms

- Fruits

- Vegetables

- Nuts

- Simple, pressed natural oils such as olive oil or coconut oil

Foods that aren't allowed under the Paleo diet are:

- Dairy Products (other than eggs)

- Refined sugars such as cane sugar, high fructose corn syrup and molasses

- Grains

- Legumes

- Processed foods or meats such as spam, most sausages, or anything where you can't tell what it started out as just by looking.

Don't get too worried, though! It's actually a lot easier than it first appears to cut the dairy and the grains out of your diet and still eat delicious, gourmet-quality food.

For example, a breakfast of mushrooms, onions and peppers in an omelet, with a grapefruit on the side fits perfectly under this diet.

For lunch you might have a ginger-apple porkchop with a salad and still be totally fine.

Dinner could be salmon, garlic zucchini, and baked pears. If you get hungry during the day, you can have a handful of almonds, a left over pork chop, and a peach without breaking your diet at all.

On the paleo diet, it isn't really *how much* you're eating, but *what* you're eating that matters. You can have as much animal protein, fruits, and non-starchy vegetables as you want.

If you are looking to lose weight quickly, it's still good to count calories to make sure you are burning more calories than you're consuming, but even if you weren't to count calories at all, as long as you're careful that the bulk of the foods you eat come from lean meats, fruits and non-starchy vegetables you will still start to slowly lose weight.

If you're thinking "I can't give up dairy and starch," don't despair!

Starchy vegetables can still be eaten on the Paleo diet, but they should be eaten in moderation. Starch is another substance that our bodies turn immediately into sugars, so keep in mind that vegetables high in starch can torpedo your weight loss on the Paleo diet if you eat too many of them.

Starchy vegetables include potatoes, sweet potatoes, beets, pumpkins, acorn or butternut squashes, corn, and parsnips. You can still indulge occasionally on these vegetables on Paleo, just be aware that they will convert to sugar in your body faster than other fruits and veggies.

These starchy vegetables might actually be good for athletes or others with high physical demands that give them serious caloric needs, but for the rest of us, treat them with caution. They shouldn't be on your daily menu.

Like all cooking, a lot of the flavor and nutritional value comes from the quality of your starting ingredients. A study recently found that many mass-produced grocery market vegetables actually have less nutrients than locally or organically-grown varieties, because the plants were not grown in nutrient-rich environments to begin with, and then not actually allowed reach full ripeness in the field! Thus, effectively cutting off their natural growing cycle.

If you get vegetables or fruits with very little flavor, it's very likely that their nutritional value is also reduced. So it's important when you're shopping to try to make sure you are buying high quality meats and produce.

For meats try to get lean, grass-fed cuts or game meats whenever possible. The normal, mass-produced, domestic meats often have additional layers of fat in them, which adds to the flavor value, but also adds to undesirable qualities like total cholesterol and fat. That being said, while it's better to get the meats that are closer to the game animals Reeja's husband hunted back in the Paleolithic, animal protein is still the basis of this diet, regardless. If you only have access to regular grocery market domesticated meats, you can be smart about the meats you pick.

Buffalo, for example, has been domesticated for much less time than cattle, and its meat is much leaner than domestic beef, while being similar in flavor. In recent years many grocery markets have started to carry it, as well.

Lamb or goat is also a reasonable substitution for the high-fat cuts of domestic beef.

Domestic beef can definitely be eaten on the Paleo diet, but just be aware that the standard, commercially available varieties have a much higher fat content than their wild ancestors, and choose lower fat cuts.

Still, if you live somewhere where you can't get specialty meats like wild-caught game or grass-fed meats don't stress out too much. Just look for leaner meats, shellfish and fish to eat on a regular basis and keep the high fat content meats for "occasional foods." Frequently-stocked lean meats, such as pork, chicken and turkey, which have been minimally processed are perfectly acceptable, as well if you can't get grass fed or wild meats.

Stay away from pre-cooked and pre-made lunch meats that already been infused with lots of sodium. By that same token, it's better to limit your intake of cured meats such as ham and bacon since they are infused with salt. You don't have to necessarily cut them out of your Paleo diet completely, but be aware of the sodium you are eating and up your number of potassium-rich fruits and vegetables on days when you eat cured meats like those. That will help you avoid losing the calcium benefit from your low-salt Paleo diet.

Fish are always a great meat to put on your Paleo menu as well, since fish have quite a few unique health benefits. For example, salmon contains Omega 3, calcium, B6, B12 and even contains a healthy amount of vitamin D.

It is still a good idea to supplement vitamin D while on the Paleo diet if you don't get a lot of time outside. While our skin has the ability to synthesize cholesterol into vitamin D, it takes a significant amount of time in the sun every single day. One of the leading Paleo Diet researchers, Loren Cordain, recommends that those of us with desk jobs or minimal time outside find a supplement that supplies at least 2,000 I.U. of vitamin D a day.

And don't forget to eat the nuts! While nuts can be high in fat and so should be eaten in moderation, they are also high in many other beneficial antioxidants, fiber, minerals and vitamins.

Don't eat them in unlimited quantity like animal protein, fruits and non-starchy vegetables on this diet, they are still a very important factor in making sure you get the dietary fiber and vitamins the human body needs.

Important note here: peanuts are actually a legume, and so are not actually a part of the Paleo pantry.

When we're talking about nuts, we're talking about actual nuts, not legumes. Peanut butter especially has been processed and had a lot of its national benefit removed. Generally speaking, the nuts included in the Paleo diet are tree nuts, such as the brazil nut, hazelnut, pecan, walnut, almond, and macadamia.

Since it's always a good idea to get the most nutritional value out of your ingredients, Omega 3 or free range eggs are also recommended over standard eggs when possible.

If you aren't sure how to jump in and starting cooking with Paleo ingredients, there are a lot of great Paleo cookbooks and recipe sites.

A couple of places to start are: http://paleomg.com/ and http://www.paleoplan.com/recipes/. Many of the introductory Paleo sites also have recipes or meal ideas. But all you really need to remember to start cooking Paleo is that you want simple, wholesome ingredients.

Throw out the sugar, milk and loaf of bread from your local market, and you're well on your way.

Eat Better to Feel Better

You may be thinking, why should I go to all this trouble to emulate Reeja's diet?

After all, it's impossible to get it *exactly* the same, because many of the animals she ate are now extinct, and the average person's access to wild foods is a lot more limited in general.

The answer to that is simple. By eating lean meats, fruits, vegetables and nuts that are easier to for your body to digest, you can lose weight, feel more energetic, and eliminate digestive problems.

Paleo also has a lot of additional health benefits in addition to being a good way to lose weight.

While it's true that the foods we can get now won't be identical to the foods Reeja's tribe hunted and gathered, but there are still a lot of benefits that come from a diet that consists of foods like Reeja's.

Let's take a look at some of the different health problems a Paleo-style eating plan can help regulate or avoid:

Diabetes

Welcome to 21st century America, the land of diabetes. The American Diabetes Association estimates that 8.3% of the population of America have diabetes. Of those, almost a third are undiagnosed.

America is a country whose blood sugar has run totally out of control. That's not surprising; think of the number of sugar-laden products that are presented to you on a daily basis. Soda? Candy? Just about anything cooked at a fast-food joint? We have a sweet tooth in this country, and it's been kicking the daylights out of our pancreases.

Diabetes is, of course, a disease in which the pancreas ceases to effectively regulate blood sugar through the production of insulin. Insulin is, if you will, the anti-sugar, the thing that keeps sugar in check.

You see, like many drugs, the human body can develop a tolerance toward insulin. (ADA)

If you constantly spam your body with sugar, then your pancreas is constantly spamming your body with insulin. Eventually, your body becomes tolerant of the insulin, making it less and less effective.

That's type II diabetes in a nutshell; prolonged and ingrained resistance to insulin.

It should not, then, be shocking that a diet that cuts out refined sugars and complex carbohydrates has a positive effect on your chance for developing or inflaming type II diabetes. By limiting those spikes in blood sugar we so love to give ourselves, we prevent the overdosing on insulin our pancreas does to deal with those spikes. As a result, it is much harder for our bodies to become tolerant of that insulin.

Furthermore, this diet helps people who have already developed diabetes maintain an even blood sugar level, often helping to eliminate the need for additional insulin. The animal protein, non-starchy fruits and vegetables don't spike blood sugars high and then bottom out in a few hours like grains or dairy products.

Osteoporosis

Osteoporosis is a pretty simple condition to understand. The word says it all: *Osteo* means "bone," and *porosis* comes from the same Latin root as "porous" or "porosity." It's porous bones.

Our bodies build and re-build our bones primarily from calcium. Now, we've cut the dairy out of your diet, but never fear! As we've discussed earlier, fruits and vegetables are actually a better source of usable calcium and vitamins than dairy products when eaten along with the high protein, lean meats that are the mainstay of the Paleo diet.

Here's the kicker, though: there's two sides to osteoporosis. On one side, there is the rate at which your body can repair wear on your bones; that's controlled by your calcium intake. The other side, though, is the acidity and salinity of your body, which cause your bones to degrade. Chugging milk will, no doubt, up your calcium levels, but it will *also* increase your levels of lactic acid. The net effect of those two substances entering your body at the same time is something of a wash with regards to osteoporosis. Sure, your bones can repair more damage, but they're also *taking* more damage.

Removing the salt and lactic acid from your diet also allows you to keep a better acid-base balance in your body, keeping the calcium in your bones from being leached out. This leads to a lower incidence of osteoporosis and other bone-loss related diseases. As a side bonus, it also helps with dental strength! The incidence of tooth loss and cavities is much lower among native populations that still practice a Paleo style diet than Western populations.

Cardiovascular problems and High Blood Pressure

People who practice a Paleo diet actually have a lower incidence of heart problems. This is partially because Paleo is low sodium, and partially because the lean meats in the Paleo diet contain a higher percentage of good fats that assist in the production of HDL's or "good cholesterol" and so can help restore heart and cardiovascular health. These beneficial fats also keep the LDL's or "bad cholesterol" from oxidizing, which allows it to coat and clog arteries.

The final reason why Paleo eating is better for cardiovascular health is because of that acid-base balance we talked about earlier. A high acid level in the body has recently been linked to high blood pressure and stoke.

That being said, while Paleo diet can be very beneficial to heart health, if you have pre-existing heart conditions, you should always seek medical supervision while changing your diet. Since you may have other medical or environmental factors to consider as well, it is important that changing to a new diet be done correctly and with the most chance for effectiveness for people with pre-existing conditions. This book is not meant as medical advice, and for those who already have serious medical problems, they should seek a doctor's assistance.

Chronic Fatigue/ Lack of Energy

Sugar is great, isn't it? You get some candy, or drink a sugary soda, and you feel great right afterward. Your body is flying high, because sugar is *so easy* for the body to turn into energy. Our bodies love getting sugar, in the short term.

The problem, of course, is that after that rush comes the crash. Thus it is that sugars and carbs actually cause us more fatigue. We get half an hour of rush, and five hours of recovery; the exchange simply isn't worth it.

The Paleo diet can help with the chronic fatigue that is often brought on by the rapid fluctuations in blood sugar cause by complex carbohydrates, such as the ones present in grain. Carbohydrate fluctuations over an extended periods of time can also lead to other chronic conditions associated with high glycemic levels such as reductions in vascular elasticity and inflammation. (Dickinson)

Vascular Inflammation

A Paleo-style diet has been shown to significantly reduce vascular inflammation among native peoples. The rate of heart attack actually approaches zero among some of the native tribes, which is virtually unheard of in Western Civilization. (European Journal of Clinical Nutrition, Burkitt)

This isn't because their blood pressure is lower than in Western populations, but their level of vascular inflammation is much, much lower.

The healthful fats in their high protein diets have insulated their vascular system from the normal causes of inflammation In fact, heart disease kills almost 1 in 4 African Americans in the US. (Center for Disease Control)

The native hunter-gatherer tribes of Africa and the African population in the US have exactly the same basic DNA structure as those living in the US. It's not a genetic issue; it's a social one. Those hunter-gatherers lead very different lifestyles, more closely following a traditional Paleo diet.

The results are easy for all to see.

Obesity

The rate of obesity among populations who practice a Paleo style diet also approaches zero.

This is, again, due to the ability of our bodies to make the most use out of the nutritional and caloric values present in the foods, which developed over millions of years.

While most native populations are very active, the total amount of exercise and the benefit the gain from physical activity has been shown to be essentially the same as Western populations. They don't sit behind a desk all day, and they are likely to get several hours of exercise through their normal daily routine, but exercise alone isn't what is keeping them trim. Now don't get me wrong. It is always best to try and fit some exercise into your day along with the diet change in order to get the maximum benefit from the Paleo diet. But researchers now agree that exercise alone can't account for all these weight differences.

Digestive Issues and Diseases

The Paleo diet is naturally high in fiber, which is instrumental in preventing and treating a surprising number of digestive problems. Lack of fiber in your normal diet can lead to heartburn, irritable bowel syndrome, constipation, indigestion, hemorrhoids, certain types of ulcer, and varicose veins, just to name a few. (Cordain, McDougall)

Auto-Immune Problems

While more extensive study needs to be done in regards to Paleo's benefits for people suffering from auto-immune disorders such as Rheumatoid arthritis, type I diabetes, and dermatitis, there is enough evidence to suggest that an interaction between the lectins contained in some grains, legumes and the intestinal wall may be at least partially to blame. The lectins contained in wheat, soybeans, and peanuts have been shown to thin the intestinal wall, and let some intestinal bacteria out into the bloodstream.

Obviously not good, right?

Well, our body has developed super antibodies to get rid of these bacteria that seep out. The only problem is, these gut bacteria contain the same structure as other tissues, and may lead the body to mistakenly attack itself. While some research has been done showing that the body can be tricked into attacking itself using food proteins found in grains, dairy, legumes, more research needs to be done on this issue before scientists can say whether a change in diet truly help with this type of disorder.

However, Auto-Immune sufferers really have very little to lose from trying this diet, and as we've shown above there are quite a few other health benefits from Paleo eating habits.

You Have Nothing to Fear

Humanity has always been resourceful. If we thought of something that would be useful, whether it was fire, fur, bow and arrow, gold, or a new disease treatment, we've found ways to make it or get our hands on it. As a result, our generation is the most resource-laden generation that has ever existed.

A typical person has more foods at their fingertips by picking up the phone or going to the grocery store than Reeja could ever have imagined.

Just for heating foods up, we have stoves, ovens, microwaves, deep fryers, grills, rotisseries, and pressure cookers. We've found ways to extract, refine, and process plants, animals, and minerals in ways that Reeja wouldn't even understand. We've found ways to make oil from vegetables, grind grains and legumes into flours or pastes, and refine sugars or even break sugar apart so it still tastes sweet, but doesn't get processed by our bodies (sucralose).

This technological and scientific progress has led to a lot of really good discoveries, making day-to-day survival much easier than it was in Reeja's time.

But as a result of all this progress, and the overall ease of getting food and resources, those living in Western countries are also one of the most obese generations, poised to overtake our parents and all previous generations in terms of lack of fitness and total weight (University of Adelaide). There's also been a spike in the "diseases of affluence," in Western civilization such as diabetes, cardiovascular disease, and hypertension. (Preventative Medicine Center)

We eat more oil, salt, grains, fatty meats, and starchy vegetables in one order of fast-food takeout than Reeja would ever get in one sitting. We eat cookies, cakes, deep fried foods that everyone admits isn't good for you. And we eat them on a regular basis, asking our bodies to deal with complex carbohydrates and fats on a daily basis. On top of that your typical Westerner doesn't get much exercise to burn off those extra calories.

Reeja and her tribe members walked and ran everywhere they went. They hunted, they fished, they dug roots and picked all kinds of vegetables and fruits. Their days were full of what we now think of as "manual labor." Which, honestly, I think most of Western culture tries to avoid.

Think about it.

Typically, if we exercise, it's more likely to be the distance between couch and kitchen, or possibly a leisurely stroll around the supermarket. According to The New York Tmes, 80% of Americans have sedentary work or "desk jobs." (Parker-Pope) If Reeja lived now, no doubt she'd be bored out of her mind. Even if she wasn't a super athlete, she got at least got hours of moderate exercise and exposure to the sun everyday. Every minute of her day was taken up with some activity to help herself and her tribe survive tomorrow and the day after.

Earlier in the book, we've talked about how changing our dietary habits to more closely resemble Reeja's eating habits can have immediate health benefits for losing weight and curing dietary problems. Reeja didn't think of the Paleo way of eating as a weight loss plan or a fad diet to be cast aside the moment she lost enough weight. This style of eating is the way humanity survived for millions of years before the industrial revolution. Since physiologically, modern humans are the same as Reeja, it makes sense that our bodies are better equipped to use the nutrients in the same foods that she ate.

Not convinced that you can leave behind your mashed potatoes, chocolate and red wine and start eating the Paleo way right now? Don't try to force yourself to give up the dishes you love cold turkey. You can transition into the Paleo diet gradually by leaving a few meals a week open to "regular style" reasonably sized meals or desserts. As long as you limit your intake of grain, dairy, legumes and sugar, to a few meals a week, you will soon see a difference.

Just be sure to watch the portion size of your "guilty pleasure" foods, like you would anything else. A little bit here or there isn't going to completely destroy your Paleo benefits as long as you the majority of your meals are still prepared in the Paleo way.

Saying you can have a free meal or dish here or there *doesn't* mean to binge on whatever you pick. For example, it doesn't mean you can sit down with a quart of ice cream and devour the whole thing as one of your "meals." But let's be honest-- that wouldn't be healthy no matter what diet regimen you decided to follow. A scoop of ice cream after one of your Paleo meals once a week probably isn't going to hurt.

When you get down to it, there are very few down sides to trying the Paleo diet– especially for people who have tried to lose weight and failed, or are struggling with health problems that regular modern medicine hasn't been able to cure. If you strip away all the modern conveniences, we are just like Reeja and her tribe. We just accumulated more toys.

Even domesticated animals are fed a mix of foods that match what they would be able to eat in the wild. Why? Because that's what they've evolved to thrive on. The elderly cat lady doesn't feed her strays carrots. Their bodies aren't equipped to digest it. You also don't feed your rabbit chicken. If you did feed the cat or the rabbit these foods that are so far removed from their natural diet, it would be extremely bad for both of them. Why is it so ridiculous when we talk about trying these type of dietary changes with our pets, and it's perfectly acceptable to do it to ourselves? Why do we think that we'll have better results when we try it with our own bodies?

The truth is that most people haven't even thought about it. After all, as long as it's not poisonous it must be ok, right? I hope if nothing else, that this book that this book has shown how wrong that line of thinking is. So now that you are aware of how bad for our bodies most of our Western diet is, what does that mean?

The thing holding most people back from trying the simple, wholesome Paleo diet is fear.

Fear of the unknown, fear of failing another diet, fear that it may be more expensive, fear that the benefits might not be quite as good as the experts say--and you'll regret having already given up all those candy bars. All of those fears can be answered really simply.

Try eating Paleo for just a week, and see how you feel afterwards. No change in diet has to be permanent. But I think you'll find that Paleo does what the dieticians say it does when followed correctly. It shouldn't be shocking that a diet like Reeja's is what our bodies are designed to digest.

It only makes sense that you'll feel better after cutting your diet back to the foods were easily available to

humans in the wild and easily digested by our bodies
due to thousands of years of evolution.

Paleo Recipe Collections

Paleo Plan Recipes:

http://www.paleoplan.com/recipes/

Grouped by different types of meals and ingredients, you'll find something for any situation. (Try the ginger brownies!)

Nom Nom Paleo:

http://nomnompaleo.com/recipeindex

Really excellent collection of recipes, this site couples the recipes with some really beautiful, top notch photography.

FastPaleo.com:

http://fastpaleo.com/

Don't have a ton of time to cook? Give Fast Paleo a look!

PaleOMG:

http://paleomg.com/

Nice collection of recipes, with holiday treats and videos too! (I just made her Sweet Potato and Apple Breakfast Patties!)

Everyday Paleo:

http://everydaypaleo.com/

An awesome, family-friendly site with recipes and lifestyle articles.

Now Available for Amazon Kindle!

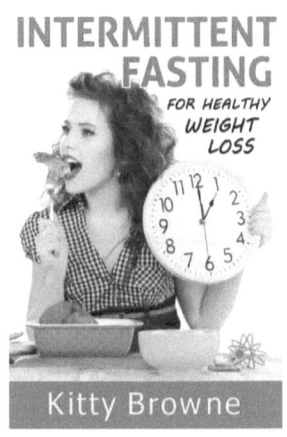

Intermittent Fasting for Healthy Weight Loss

The Green Juice Revolution

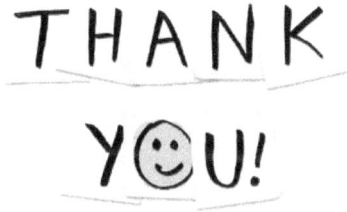

Thanks for Reading!

If you enjoyed this introduction to the world of intermittent fasting, please consider telling a friend about this book and leaving us some positive feedback on Amazon.com!

We sincerely appreciate all feedback from readers.

To learn more, visit KittyBrowne.com

Bibliography

Cordain, Loren, PhD. The Paleo Diet, 2002,2011.

Joulwan, Melissa; Petrucci, Kellyann Living Paleo for Dummies, December 2012.

Paleolithic Diet,
http://en.wikipedia.org/wiki/Paleolithic_diet

The Paleolithic Diet Nutrition page,
http://www.paleodiet.com/

Are Whole Grains Making us fat?
http://www.thesweetbeet.com/whole-grains/

Starchy Vegetable List
http://diabetes.about.com/od/nutrition/a/List-Of-Starchy-Vegetables.htm

Harvard Health. "Calcium and Milk: Strong Bones with Vegetables"
http://www.hsph.harvard.edu/nutritionsource/calcium-and-milk/

Crinion, Walter J. ND. "Organic Foods Contain Higher Levels of Nutrients", http://www.altmedrev.com/publications/15/1/4.pdf

Center for Disease Control, "Heart Disease Rates in the US by Ethnicity" http://www.cdc.gov/heartdisease/facts.htm

Wolf, Robb, The Paleo Solution: The original Human Diet, 2011.

Lindeberg, Staffan; Cordain, Loren; Eaton, S. Boyd (September 2003). "Biological and Clinical

Potential of a Palaeolithic Diet". Journal of Nutritional and Environmental Medicine 13 (3): 149–60.

Kligler, Benjamin & Lee, Roberta A. (eds.) (2004). "Paleolithic diet". Integrative medicine.

Eaton, S.Boyd; Cordain, Loren; Lindeberg, Staffan (2002). "Evolutionary Health Promotion: A

Consideration of Common Counterarguments". Preventive Medicine 34 (2): 119–23.

Challem, Jack, "Paleolithic Nutrition: Your Future is in Your Dietary Past". Nutrition Reporter. 1997.

http://web.archive.org/web/20080616145456/http://www.nutritionreporter.com/stone_age_diet.html

Schocker, Lauren, "Surprisingly Calcium-Rich Foods That Aren't Milk", Huffington Post 4/25/2012.

Centers for Disease Control and Prevention, "Fruits and Vegetables" http://www.cdc.gov/nutrition/everyone/fruitsvegetables/

Quinn, Neely. "Is Paleo Safe for Diabetics," http://www.paleoplan.com/2012/08-17/is-paleo-safe-for-diabetics/

Tiel, Sharon, www.LiveStrong.com, "Buffalo vs. Beef" http://www.livestrong.com/article/372112-buffalo-meat-versus-beef-nutrition/

King, Sandra, www.LiveStrong.com "Nutritional Value of Goat Meat Compared to Other Meats"

http://www.livestrong.com/article/328432-nutritional-value-of-goat-meat-compared-to-other-meats/

Cordain, Loren, http://thepaleodiet.com/nut-fatty-acid-composition/

Klonloff, David, "The Beneficial Effects of a Paleolithic Diet on Type 2 Diabetes and Other Risk Factors for Cardiovascular Disease" J Diabetes Sci Technol. 2009 November; 3(6): 1229–1232

L Cordain, SB Eaton, J Brand Miller, N Mann and K Hill, European Journal of Clinical Nutrition: "The paradoxical nature of hunter-gatherer diets: meat-based, yet non-atherogenic," (2002) 56, Suppl 1, S42–S52

Herman Pontzer, David A. Raichlen, Brian M. Wood, Audax Z. P. Mabulla,Susan B. Racette, Frank W. Marlowe, "Hunter-Gatherer Energetics and Human Obesity", 2012.

Loren Cordain, S Boyd Eaton, Anthony Sebastian, Neil Mann, Staffan Lindeberg, Bruce A Watkins, James H O'Keefe, and Janette Brand-Miller, "Origins and evolution of the Western diet: health implications for the 21st century," http://ajcn.nutrition.org/content/81/2/341.full.pdf

Scott Dickinson, Dale P Hancock, Peter Petocz, Antonio Ceriello, and Jennie Brand-Miller,

"High–glycemic index carbohydrate increases nuclear factor-?B activation in mononuclear cells of young, lean healthy subjects", American Society for Clinical Nutrition. 2008.

H.C. Trowell and D.P Burkitt, *Western Diseases: Their Emergence and Prevention*, 1981.

Dr. McDougall's Health and Medical Center, "Constipation, Hemorrhoids, Varicose Veins", 2013. http://www.drmcdougall.com/med_constipation.html

University of Adelaide. "Gen X overtaking baby boomers on obesity." ScienceDaily, 1 Nov. 2012. Web. 4 Jul. 2013.

American Diabetes Association, "Diabetes Statistics," http://www.diabetes.org/diabetes-basics/diabetes-statistics/

Gedgaudas, Nora T. CNS, CNT. "Primal Body, Primal Mind: Beyond the Paleo Diet for Total Health and a Longer Life." 2011.

Preventive Medicine Center, "Diet and Disease," http://www.thepmc.org/2009/12/library-diet-and-disease/